UNDERSTANDING

MESOTHERAPY

FOR BEGINNERS

Unlocking The Secrets Of Non-Surgical Aesthetic Treatments For Skin Rejuvenation, Fat Loss, And Cellulite Reduction

DR. ALICIA SONYA

CONTENTS

DISCLAIMER

The information provided in this book is for educational and informational purposes only and is not intended as medical advice, diagnosis, or treatment. Always consult with a qualified healthcare professional before beginning any therapy, practice, or lifestyle change.

The author and publisher of this book make no representations or warranties regarding the accuracy, applicability, or completeness of the content presented. While every effort has been made to ensure the information provided is accurate and up-to-date, the field of health and wellness is constantly evolving, and the reader is advised to use discretion and seek professional guidance as needed.

This book contains references to individuals, products, websites, organizations, or other entities solely for informational purposes. The author and publisher do not endorse, sponsor, or affiliate with any of these references, nor do they receive any benefit from their inclusion. The mention of any names, trademarks, or products does not imply any association or endorsement.

The use of this book is solely at the reader's discretion. Neither the author nor the publisher shall be held liable for any damages, loss, or injury resulting from the use or misuse of the information contained herein.

ABOUT THIS BOOK

Understanding mesotherapy For Beginners "offers an essential resource for those seeking to understand and experience the transformative potential of mesotherapy, a minimally invasive procedure known for its skin, fat loss, and cellulite treatment benefits. This book delves deeply into the origins and mechanisms behind mesotherapy, explaining its role within the field of aesthetics and distinguishing it from other treatment options. By exploring the science behind mesotherapy, this book helps readers grasp how this treatment rejuvenates and contours the skin and body through targeted ingredients and specialized techniques.

A solid understanding of skin and body aesthetics lays the foundation for effective mesotherapy treatments. Readers will gain insight into skin anatomy, fat storage, and the process behind cellulite formation, along with considerations specific to various skin types. This essential knowledge assists readers in identifying which areas of their body are suitable for mesotherapy and understanding how mesotherapy compares to traditional anti-aging and contouring methods.

When it comes to skin rejuvenation, this guide provides detailed explanations of the specific goals mesotherapy addresses, from brightening to hydration and anti-aging. By introducing readers to the common ingredients used in skin mesotherapy, along with techniques for treating areas like the face and neck, this book enables a comprehensive understanding of the rejuvenation process. Practical tips on pre- and post-treatment care further empower readers to maintain and optimize their results.

Mesotherapy's role in fat loss and cellulite reduction is equally significant, with sections dedicated to the body's target areas for these treatments. By outlining the ingredients and formulations used for fat-burning and cellulite management, this book offers an in-depth look at the step-by-step process. Clear information on treatment frequency, expected outcomes, and realistic expectations make this guide an invaluable reference for anyone considering mesotherapy for body contouring.

For those interested in mesotherapy's technical side, this guide explains the different methods and tools used, such as micro-injections, derma rollers, and needle-free techniques. Readers learn how to choose the most appropriate methods based on their goals, while the emphasis on safety and hygiene practices ensures a safe and effective experience. Furthermore, it details recent advancements in application technology that continue to elevate the field of mesotherapy.

In terms of ingredients, the guide provides an extensive breakdown of common substances used in mesotherapy, including those for skin brightening, hydration, and fat burning. This book underscores the importance of quality in product sourcing and helps readers learn how to interpret ingredient lists, a crucial skill for informed and safe treatment choices. The guidance on personalized formulations also highlights how each treatment can be tailored to individual needs.

Preparing for a mesotherapy session can be a significant part of the experience, and this book offers insights into the consultation process, pre-treatment do's and don'ts, and ways to manage anxiety or discomfort. Practical questions to ask a practitioner ensure that readers are well-prepared, while sections on cost factors and treatment plans give a realistic view of what to expect financially.

Aftercare is critical to achieving optimal results, and this guide dedicates a section to post-treatment care, addressing common side effects and providing tips on prolonging the benefits of mesotherapy. From skincare routines to the timing of follow-up treatments, readers receive comprehensive advice on how to take charge of their recovery process.

For those with questions or concerns, this book includes an accessible FAQ section addressing the safety and effectiveness of mesotherapy, variations in individual results, and the implications of missing a session. Additionally, readers learn how mesotherapy can be combined with other aesthetic treatments for enhanced results.

Finally, selecting a qualified practitioner is fundamental, and the guide provides criteria for evaluating credentials, clinic standards, and practitioner expertise.

By guiding readers through questions and considerations for customizing a treatment plan, this book fosters informed decision-making, helping readers set realistic expectations and choose a provider who aligns with their aesthetic goals. This comprehensive guide is an invaluable asset for those ready to explore the innovative, multi-faceted world of mesotherapy.

CHAPTER ONE

Introduction To Mesotherapy

Mesotherapy is a minimally invasive procedure where a series of injections deliver vitamins, enzymes, hormones, and plant extracts into the skin to rejuvenate it and remove excess fat.

Developed in France in the 1950s, mesotherapy initially aimed at pain relief, but over time, practitioners discovered its aesthetic benefits, especially for skin rejuvenation, fat loss, and hair growth. The treatment uses micro-injections to administer active substances just beneath the surface of the skin, which can vary depending on the treatment's goal, from revitalizing skin to reducing localized fat.

Practitioners use tiny needles to inject targeted solutions into the mesodermal layer of skin, which is the middle layer between fat and tissue. This technique allows substances to reach where topical creams cannot, stimulating the body's natural healing processes and addressing concerns like wrinkles, fine lines, and stubborn fat deposits. These ingredients can include hyaluronic acid, peptides, or natural extracts designed to nourish and revitalize the skin or dissolve fat cells.

Mesotherapy sessions are typically short, lasting 20 to 30 minutes, depending on the area and purpose. Results vary by individual, with many noticing improvements in skin texture or reduced cellulite after just a few treatments. It's a versatile option for non-surgical skin improvement, and patients can generally resume daily activities shortly after the procedure with minimal downtime.

Understanding Mesotherapy And Its Origins

The practice of mesotherapy was pioneered by French doctor Michel Pistor in the 1950s, who initially used it for pain management. As he observed its positive effects on various conditions, including blood circulation and skin quality, mesotherapy began to expand into different fields. Over time, it became especially popular within the beauty industry due to its potential for targeted treatment, offering a less invasive approach to addressing common aesthetic issues.

In the early days, mesotherapy mostly involved herbal and pharmaceutical substances, combined with mechanical stimulation to improve circulation and relieve pain.

Today, however, the procedure has evolved significantly, incorporating advanced compounds and specialized equipment. Modern mesotherapy uses techniques derived from dermatology, aesthetics, and pharmacology, making it a highly specialized procedure that requires a certified professional for safe and effective treatment.

The popularity of mesotherapy has surged due to its adaptability and wide application range, from anti-aging treatments to fat reduction.

Various countries have embraced mesotherapy, developing unique adaptations to suit their patients' needs. Though initially met with skepticism, it is now recognized as a viable option for those seeking non-surgical aesthetic enhancements.

How It Works: The Science Behind Mesotherapy

Mesotherapy works by delivering active compounds directly into the skin's mesodermal layer, where cellular regeneration, fat metabolism, and skin repair processes occur.

The micro-injections contain a mix of nutrients and medications tailored to individual needs, stimulating the skin's natural repair processes.

This technique bypasses the skin's surface barrier, allowing active ingredients to penetrate deeper than creams or serums, providing faster, more noticeable results.

The injected substances can vary widely depending on the treatment's purpose. For example, anti-aging mesotherapy may use antioxidants, hyaluronic acid, and vitamins to boost collagen production and hydrate the skin.

For fat reduction, mesotherapy injections might include substances that break down fat cells, which are then naturally eliminated by the body. The compounds promote micro-circulation, cellular turnover, and metabolic stimulation, contributing to the desired effects.

The needle used is extremely thin, allowing for multiple tiny injections in a single area without significant pain or bruising. Each injection is precisely placed to ensure optimal distribution of active ingredients. The localized delivery is part of what makes mesotherapy so effective, as the substances target the exact area where rejuvenation or fat breakdown is desired.

Comparing Mesotherapy To Other Aesthetic Treatments

Mesotherapy stands out among aesthetic treatments for its precision and versatility, offering advantages over treatments like botox, fillers, and liposuction. Unlike botox, which focuses primarily on wrinkle reduction by temporarily paralyzing muscles, mesotherapy rejuvenates the skin through nourishing injections.

Similarly, fillers add volume, while mesotherapy improves skin health overall by stimulating collagen production, hydration, and elasticity.

Compared to liposuction, which is a surgical procedure for fat removal, mesotherapy is non-surgical and less invasive, making it a more accessible choice for people seeking to target stubborn fat pockets without extensive downtime.

Liposuction involves longer recovery and potential scarring, whereas mesotherapy's micro-injections require minimal downtime and are generally safe for localized fat reduction in areas like the chin, thighs, or abdomen.

In contrast with treatments like micro-needling, which relies on tiny needles to boost collagen production, mesotherapy delivers a personalized blend of nutrients directly into the skin, providing more immediate visible results for hydration, anti-aging, and fat breakdown. Patients can also combine mesotherapy with other treatments, making it a flexible option for those looking to enhance their appearance without committing to surgery.

Key Benefits Of Mesotherapy For Skin, Fat Loss, And Cellulite

Mesotherapy offers a range of benefits tailored to different aesthetic goals. For skin rejuvenation, the treatment enhances hydration, firmness, and radiance by delivering a blend of hyaluronic acid, vitamins, and antioxidants directly into the skin layers. This process addresses fine lines, improves skin tone, and restores a youthful glow, making it especially popular for aging or sun-damaged skin.

When it comes to fat loss, mesotherapy can help with spot reduction by breaking down fat cells in targeted areas like the abdomen, thighs, and chin.

The active compounds, usually including fat-dissolving agents, are injected into the problem areas, where they act on fat cells, breaking them down so they can be naturally flushed from the body. This approach is beneficial for individuals who struggle with localized fat deposits that don't respond well to diet or exercise.

Mesotherapy is also effective for reducing the appearance of cellulite by improving blood circulation and breaking down fibrous connective tissues under the skin. The injections help to smooth and tighten the skin over time, reducing dimpling and uneven textures commonly associated with cellulite. For best results, patients may need multiple sessions, but many report smoother skin and noticeable improvement in cellulite within a few treatments.

Types Of Mesotherapy Treatments Available Today

Mesotherapy can be tailored to address various concerns, with types ranging from anti-aging and skin brightening to fat loss and hair restoration. Anti-aging mesotherapy, for instance, includes ingredients like vitamins, amino acids, and hyaluronic acid to boost collagen and elasticity, softening fine lines and improving overall skin texture. This type is common for facial rejuvenation, giving the skin a youthful glow.

Another popular type is lipolytic mesotherapy, designed specifically for fat and cellulite reduction. This involves injecting fat-dissolving substances, often combined with circulation-enhancing agents, to target stubborn fat areas and cellulite. Lipolytic mesotherapy is frequently used on areas like the thighs, abdomen, and arms, helping to reshape and tone the body without invasive procedures.

Hair mesotherapy is increasingly popular for those dealing with thinning hair or hair loss.

This involves injecting nutrients directly into the scalp to stimulate hair follicles, increase blood circulation, and encourage new hair growth.

By nourishing the roots, hair mesotherapy can strengthen existing hair and promote growth, making it a non-surgical option for people with mild to moderate hair loss.

32

CHAPTER TWO

Understanding The Skin And Body In Aesthetics

In aesthetics, understanding the skin's structure is essential for effective treatments like mesotherapy. The skin has three main layers: the epidermis, dermis, and hypodermis (subcutaneous tissue). The epidermis is the outermost layer that protects against environmental factors, while the dermis contains collagen and elastin, which keep skin firm and elastic.

The hypodermis stores fat and provides insulation. This complex structure changes as we age, with collagen loss, slower cell turnover, and reduced elasticity leading to visible signs of aging, such as fine lines and sagging.

Skin changes over time due to both intrinsic factors, like genetics and age, and extrinsic factors, such as sun exposure, pollution, and lifestyle choices. UV exposure, in particular, can break down collagen fibers, accelerating aging. In addition, repetitive muscle movements can cause expression lines, while loss of moisture leads to a dull complexion. Understanding these aging factors helps in identifying targeted areas for aesthetic treatments to restore and rejuvenate the skin.

Mesotherapy works by delivering active ingredients directly to the dermis, addressing specific issues like skin hydration, elasticity, and pigmentation.

The technique involves micro-injections that allow for precise application in areas needing improvement. By targeting the skin's deeper layers, mesotherapy can aid in replenishing essential nutrients, stimulating collagen, and improving blood circulation to rejuvenate the skin. For beginners, understanding this anatomy and aging process ensures treatments are both targeted and effective.

Basics Of Skin Anatomy And Aging Factors

The skin's structure consists of the outer epidermis, the middle dermis, and the lower hypodermis. The epidermis, with multiple cell layers, acts as a barrier, while the dermis contains collagen, elastin, and blood vessels that support skin strength and resilience. The hypodermis, or subcutaneous layer, is mainly fat and connective tissue, providing insulation and cushioning. Together, these layers protect, hydrate, and maintain overall skin health.

Aging affects these layers differently, often beginning in the dermis, where collagen and elastin fibers gradually break down. This structural loss leads to sagging, lines, and reduced skin thickness. Other aging factors include slower cell regeneration in the epidermis and decreased fat storage in the hypodermis, which can cause hollowing and fine lines.

External factors, like UV radiation and pollution, accelerate these changes, causing pigmentation, rough texture, and overall aging.

By understanding these layers and factors, practitioners can use mesotherapy to target specific needs, from hydration and collagen restoration to pigmentation correction. Mesotherapy's blend of vitamins, minerals, and hyaluronic acid helps combat aging at the cellular level, directly reaching the dermis where it stimulates collagen and elastin production. This makes it an effective choice for managing aging skin compared to surface-only treatments.

Fat Storage, Cellulite Formation, And Body Contours

Fat storage is a natural body function, primarily located in the hypodermis. Genetics, diet, and lifestyle influence where and how much fat accumulates, often leading to stubborn areas like the abdomen, thighs, and hips. Over time, the fat cells may clump together and push against the connective tissues, creating an uneven surface appearance known as cellulite, which affects body contours.

Cellulite occurs when fat deposits press against connective tissue bands under the skin, causing a dimpled or lumpy texture. Hormones, circulation issues, and lifestyle choices can worsen their appearance.

Mesotherapy treatments target these fat pockets and cellulite by injecting fat-dissolving agents, which break down localized fat, improve circulation and encourage collagen production, resulting in smoother contours.

Mesotherapy offers a minimally invasive approach to body contouring and cellulite reduction. The injected ingredients stimulate the breakdown of fat cells, allowing the body to naturally process and eliminate them. Treatments are typically spread over several sessions for gradual improvement in targeted areas. This method allows for precision in contouring and smoothing, addressing stubborn fat and cellulite with minimal downtime.

Common Skin Issues And Areas For Mesotherapy Application

Mesotherapy addresses various skin concerns, including dehydration, fine lines, pigmentation, and dullness. Common areas treated include the face, neck, décolleté, and hands, where aging signs tend to appear more prominently. Each area has unique needs; for example, the under-eye region may require hydration, while the cheeks benefit from volume and firmness.

In addition to facial areas, mesotherapy is popular for targeting cellulite and loose skin on the body. Typical areas for body treatments include the thighs, abdomen, and arms, where fat deposits and cellulite formation commonly occur. Mesotherapy injections here may include fat-dissolving ingredients to reduce localized fat, while vitamins and minerals aid in skin tightening and overall tone.

Mesotherapy uses specific cocktails tailored to the issue at hand, like hyaluronic acid for hydration, antioxidants for skin repair, and peptides for collagen stimulation. The technique allows for deep and even distribution, making it ideal for spot-treating skin concerns across different body areas. Results appear gradually, with sessions spaced over weeks for optimal outcomes.

Skin Types And Considerations For Mesotherapy

Understanding skin type is essential before mesotherapy, as the treatment approach varies between oily, dry, combination, and sensitive skin. Each type has unique characteristics, such as oil production and sensitivity levels, which affect the treatment's outcome. For instance, oily skin may need purifying agents, while dry skin benefits from added hydration and nutrients.

Sensitive skin requires a cautious approach, with gentle ingredients and minimal needle exposure to avoid irritation. In contrast, mature skin may require a higher concentration of active ingredients like peptides and antioxidants to combat aging signs. Combination skin, with both oily and dry zones, may need customized treatment in different areas for balanced results.

Practitioners assess each client's skin type, lifestyle, and specific concerns to create a personalized mesotherapy plan. The goal is to provide the right nutrients and hydration without overwhelming the skin. Adjusting the ingredients based on skin type ensures effective and safe results, especially for beginners looking to rejuvenate their skin with minimal side effects.

Mesotherapy Vs. Traditional Anti-Aging Methods

Traditional anti-aging treatments often include topical creams, serums, and invasive procedures like facelifts. While topical products are non-invasive, they only penetrate the surface, limiting their effectiveness. In contrast, mesotherapy delivers nutrients directly into the dermis, bypassing the skin's protective barrier for faster and more targeted results.

Compared to more invasive methods, mesotherapy is minimally invasive, with fewer side effects and little downtime. Instead of surgical lifting, it uses micro-injections of active ingredients to tighten and rejuvenate skin from within. This makes it appealing to those seeking natural-looking results without undergoing major procedures or extended recovery.

Mesotherapy provides versatility and customization that many traditional methods lack. Treatments can be tailored with different vitamins, minerals, and peptides to address specific aging concerns. This targeted approach makes mesotherapy a valuable alternative, especially for those looking for effective results with a gentle, customizable treatment plan.

CHAPTER THREE

Mesotherapy For Skin Rejuvenation

Overview Of Skin Rejuvenation Goals

Mesotherapy for skin rejuvenation aims to improve the skin's appearance by addressing common concerns such as fine lines, wrinkles, uneven skin tone, and dehydration.

The process involves injecting a blend of vitamins, minerals, and other nourishing substances directly into the mesoderm—the middle layer of skin—where they can promote cellular regeneration and hydration. The primary goal is to revitalize the skin and restore a youthful glow without invasive procedures like facelifts.

Common Ingredients Used In Skin Mesotherapy

The formulations used in mesotherapy can vary based on the specific needs of the skin but typically include ingredients like hyaluronic acid, vitamins (such as B and C), amino acids, and antioxidants. Hyaluronic acid helps retain moisture and provides plumpness, while vitamins nourish and protect the skin from oxidative stress. Other components, like phosphatidylcholine and deoxycholic acid, can help break down fat and improve the contour of the face, creating a more sculpted look.

Techniques For Mesotherapy On The Face And Neck

To perform mesotherapy on the face and neck, practitioners usually employ a fine needle or a specialized mesotherapy device to inject the solution into targeted areas. Treatments typically begin with cleansing the skin and applying a topical anesthetic to minimize discomfort. The injections are made in a series of small amounts at various depths, focusing on areas that show signs of aging or unevenness. Sessions typically last between 30 to 60 minutes, and multiple sessions are often recommended for optimal results.

Expected Results And Realistic Timelines

Patients can expect to see improvements in skin texture, hydration, and overall radiance after just one session. However, for more significant results, a series of treatments (usually spaced a few weeks apart) is advisable. Most people start to notice more pronounced effects around the fourth or fifth session, as collagen production increases and the skin becomes more resilient. It's important to manage expectations, as results may vary based on individual skin conditions and treatment adherence.

Pre- And Post-Treatment Care Tips For Skin Health

Before mesotherapy, it's crucial to prepare the skin by avoiding sun exposure, alcohol, and blood-thinning medications for a few days. Hydrating the skin and maintaining a balanced diet can also enhance results. After treatment, patients should avoid strenuous exercise, excessive sun exposure, and hot baths for at least 48 hours to prevent irritation. Using a gentle cleanser and applying a hydrating serum can support the healing process and prolong results.

CHAPTER FOUR

Mesotherapy For Fat Loss And Cellulite Reduction

Mesotherapy is a minimally invasive cosmetic procedure targeting localized fat deposits and cellulite. Using a series of small injections, it delivers vitamins, enzymes, hormones, and plant extracts directly into the mesoderm (middle layer of the skin). This technique is intended to dissolve fat cells, enhance blood flow, and improve lymphatic drainage, all of which help to diminish fat and smoothen the appearance of cellulite. It's most effective for people with mild to moderate fat deposits, especially in areas that resist diet and exercise.

The mesotherapy procedure itself begins with marking the targeted area and then applying a numbing cream for comfort. After the skin is prepared, a series of injections are made, usually with a very fine needle or a specialized mesotherapy injection gun, to deliver the customized blend of fat-dissolving solutions. Each session lasts around 20-30 minutes depending on the area being treated, and most patients report minimal discomfort due to the numbing.

It is important to note that mesotherapy is not a solution for significant weight loss but rather for contouring specific areas. Visible improvements in treated areas, such as reduced circumference and smoother skin, typically become noticeable after 2-4 sessions. For best results, a treatment plan often includes a few initial sessions spaced one to two weeks apart, with maintenance sessions every few months as needed. Results are gradual, as it takes time for the body to flush out the dissolved fat cells.

Target Areas For Fat Loss With Mesotherapy

Mesotherapy can be used to target multiple areas of the body where stubborn fat tends to accumulate. Commonly treated areas include the abdomen, thighs, buttocks, upper arms, and even under the chin. These areas are chosen for their tendency to store excess fat and their resistance to traditional weight-loss methods, making mesotherapy a useful addition to other lifestyle changes.

The treatment is also ideal for areas that need subtle contouring rather than major volume reduction. For example, under the chin and jawline, mesotherapy can help to achieve a smoother, more defined profile. Mesotherapy's ability to target specific spots without affecting surrounding tissues makes it an appealing choice for sculpting in smaller areas like the inner thighs or love handles.

For each targeted area, the injection dosage and treatment frequency are tailored to the specific body part's needs and the amount of fat present. Small, precise injections allow for customization in each session, ensuring the solution reaches precisely where it's needed. Multiple sessions may be necessary to see a reduction, with results developing over time as the fat-dissolving process progresses.

Key Ingredients And Solutions For Fat-Burning

Mesotherapy uses a blend of carefully chosen ingredients, each contributing to fat breakdown and skin tightening. Phosphatidylcholine and deoxycholate are two of the most common ingredients due to their ability to dissolve fat cells. These ingredients break down the fat membranes, allowing the body to process and eliminate them naturally. Additionally, ingredients like hyaluronic acid can improve hydration, while caffeine stimulates circulation and metabolism in the area.

Vitamins and minerals, including vitamin C and B-complex vitamins, are often included to support collagen production and improve the elasticity of the treated skin.

Natural extracts, like artichoke or horsetail, can enhance the effects by reducing fluid retention and promoting skin tightening. Some solutions may also include amino acids, which can aid in the metabolism of fatty acids, helping the body to flush out toxins and fat more efficiently.

Before the procedure, the professional assesses the client's skin type and body fat composition to determine the most appropriate solution. A patch test may be conducted to prevent allergic reactions. The formulation varies depending on the treatment goal—whether it's fat reduction or cellulite management—ensuring that each client receives a personalized approach for optimal results.

Steps Involved In Treating Cellulite With Mesotherapy

Cellulite treatment with mesotherapy involves several structured steps, starting with a thorough consultation. During this consultation, the practitioner assesses the cellulite's grade, which ranges from mild to severe, to customize the solution. After a numbing agent is applied, the professional uses fine injections to target dimpled skin areas, injecting the solution just beneath the skin's surface. This localized approach breaks down the fat beneath the skin, reduces fluid buildup, and stimulates collagen production, resulting in smoother skin texture.

Injections are placed strategically across the treatment area, covering each dimple and its surrounding regions to evenly distribute the solution. This method allows the ingredients to work on breaking down fat clusters and improving microcirculation in the region. Clients may feel slight tingling during the procedure, but the numbing cream minimizes discomfort.

Following the procedure, the body gradually absorbs the broken-down fat cells, with visible results appearing over a few weeks. Redness or mild bruising may occur but typically subsides within a few days.

The number of sessions depends on the cellulite's severity, but generally, 3-6 sessions are recommended for optimal smoothing and firming results.

Treatment Frequency And Anticipated Results

The frequency of mesotherapy sessions depends on the treatment goals and the client's unique needs. For most fat-reduction treatments, sessions are spaced about one to two weeks apart to allow time for the body to process and eliminate fat.

After 2-4 sessions, clients may start noticing reductions in fat volume, although full results are often seen after 6-8 sessions for more substantial areas.

When treating cellulite, results may take longer, and 3-6 sessions are usually required to see smoother skin. Maintenance treatments every 3-6 months help sustain the effects, especially for areas prone to cellulite reformation. A combination of treatments, lifestyle changes, and regular physical activity can enhance the results and prolong their duration.

While mesotherapy offers visible results, it's important to remember that it is a gradual process. Results vary from person to person, and individual response times will depend on skin type, age, and metabolic rate. Generally, clients experience long-lasting improvements, though additional sessions may be necessary to maintain the contoured appearance.

Managing Expectations: What Mesotherapy Can And Can't Do For Fat And Cellulite

Mesotherapy is effective in targeting stubborn, localized fat and smoothing out mild to moderate cellulite. However, it's not a weight-loss solution and does not provide results comparable to liposuction or other surgical methods for those seeking major reductions. Mesotherapy is best suited for body contouring, allowing people to enhance specific areas rather than achieve significant overall weight loss.

It's important to approach mesotherapy with realistic expectations. While it can lead to notable improvements in fat reduction and skin texture, results are generally moderate and are intended to complement a healthy lifestyle, not replace it. The body naturally eliminates the broken-down fat over time, so patience is key, as the process does not provide instant results.

Clients should be aware of potential side effects, such as mild bruising, swelling, or sensitivity, especially in sensitive skin areas. Following post-care instructions—such as staying hydrated and avoiding direct sunlight on treated areas—can support quicker recovery and maximize outcomes. Mesotherapy offers promising benefits when combined with proper self-care and realistic goals.

CHAPTER FIVE

Mesotherapy Techniques And Injection Methods

Mesotherapy involves several injection methods to deliver vitamins, enzymes, hormones, and plant extracts into the middle layer of the skin (mesoderm) for skin rejuvenation, fat reduction, and overall wellness.

The primary techniques include micro-injections, derma rollers, and no-needle methods. Micro-injections use fine needles to precisely target specific areas with small amounts of mesotherapy solution, ideal for skin rejuvenation and fat reduction. Dermarollers, equipped with tiny needles on a roller, are typically rolled over larger areas, allowing solutions to penetrate more evenly. No-needle methods, often using iontophoresis or electroporation, deliver mesotherapy ingredients without needles, using electric currents or ultrasound to push products into the skin.

Choosing the right mesotherapy technique depends on individual goals and tolerance for needles. For those targeting localized fat reduction or deep skin issues, micro-injections are effective but may cause mild discomfort.

For larger areas or beginners hesitant about needles, derma rollers provide a less invasive way to stimulate skin healing and absorption, though they may not deliver as deep results as injections. No-needle options are especially popular among those looking to avoid any injection pain or recovery time, though they tend to have less intense effects and may require more sessions.

Maintaining strict safety and hygiene is crucial in mesotherapy, particularly when using needles. Practitioners should use sterilized equipment, wear gloves, and disinfect the treatment area to prevent infection. For DIY enthusiasts, thoroughly sanitize your hands and equipment, follow all instructions for sterilization, and only use reputable, licensed products.

Understanding the differences between injection and non-injection methods and following recommended hygiene practices ensures safe, effective treatment.

Overview Of Injection Techniques: Micro-Injections, Dermarollers, And No-Needle Methods

Micro-injections involve the use of very fine needles to inject active ingredients directly into targeted skin layers, ensuring deep penetration of nutrients and fat-dissolving substances. This technique allows precision in areas like the face, neck, and even small pockets of body fat. Due to the depth of penetration, micro-injections are highly effective, though they can cause mild discomfort and require post-treatment care to reduce any swelling or bruising.

Dermarollers, which are handheld tools with numerous tiny needles on a roller, are moved over the skin's surface to create micro-channels.

This method encourages collagen production and enhances the absorption of mesotherapy solutions across broader skin areas, ideal for areas like the face, arms, and thighs. While derma rollers don't reach the same depth as micro-injections, they provide significant rejuvenation benefits and are suitable for at-home treatments with proper hygiene.

The no-needle method is the least invasive, using technologies like iontophoresis (electrical currents) or electroporation (ultrasound waves) to push nutrients into the skin without puncturing it. This technique is particularly useful for clients with low pain tolerance or those aiming for general skin health. Though painless, no-needle mesotherapy may deliver more superficial results and typically requires multiple sessions for noticeable effects.

Choosing The Right Technique For Your Goals

When selecting a mesotherapy technique, start by defining your goals. If you're aiming for facial rejuvenation and a fresh, lifted look, micro-injections are a popular choice, offering fast, precise results by reaching the deeper skin layers.

Those looking for a general glow or gradual skin improvement might prefer derma rollers, which provide a gentle yet effective approach that can be safely done at home. For clients wary of needles, the no-needle method offers a way to hydrate and brighten skin without any puncturing, though it usually requires more sessions.

Your pain tolerance and comfort level with needles should also guide your choice. Micro-injections and derma rollers involve some mild discomfort, especially for first-time users, but the benefits in collagen stimulation and nutrient absorption make them worth considering for long-term results. If you're entirely needle-averse, opt for no-needle mesotherapy—ideal for individuals looking to start slow and build confidence with the mesotherapy process.

Consider the frequency and budget when choosing a technique. Micro-injections, though more intensive, can often deliver longer-lasting results and may require fewer treatments. Dermarollers and no-needle techniques may need more consistent, regular treatments to achieve desired effects, but they come with the advantage of minimal downtime and generally lower initial costs, making them accessible for those just beginning with mesotherapy.

Safety And Hygiene Practices In Mesotherapy

Safety and hygiene are vital in mesotherapy, especially due to the skin's exposure to needles or other delivery methods. Before any mesotherapy session, practitioners should clean and sterilize all equipment, disinfect the treatment area, and wash their hands thoroughly. Patients undergoing the treatment should ensure the practitioner uses sealed, sterile syringes and follows professional standards to minimize any risk of infection.

If performing mesotherapy at home with a derma roller or no-needle device, take care to clean your tools thoroughly before and after use. Begin by disinfecting the derma roller with alcohol and allowing it to dry before rolling it across the skin. For no-needle devices, follow manufacturer guidelines for cleaning and storing to prevent contamination. After the treatment, avoid touching or applying any makeup on the treated area for at least 12 hours, as the skin is highly receptive during this time.

In addition to cleanliness, be cautious about skin reactions and always conduct a patch test with new mesotherapy products.

Individuals with sensitive skin may experience mild redness or irritation after mesotherapy, which is usually temporary. Keep an antiseptic or gentle soothing gel on hand to reduce redness, and contact a medical professional if irritation persists or intensifies.

Differences Between Injection And Non-Injection Methods

Injection-based mesotherapy methods, such as micro-injections, involve needles to penetrate the skin's deeper layers, directly delivering active ingredients into the mesoderm. This technique is highly effective for localized issues, like fat pockets or deep skin rejuvenation, and allows practitioners to use a lower dosage of product with a more targeted impact. Due to the direct penetration, micro-injections often yield faster results but come with a bit of post-treatment downtime, such as minor swelling or bruising.

Non-injection methods, like derma rollers or no-needle devices, involve surface-level treatments that encourage gradual absorption through microchannels or electric currents. Dermarollers, with tiny needles, stimulate collagen and improve product absorption but are less invasive than direct injections. No-needle options are entirely non-invasive, making them ideal for sensitive skin types and those averse to needles, though they often require multiple sessions for noticeable results due to the limited penetration depth.

Choosing between injection and non-injection methods depends on the desired results, skin sensitivity, and tolerance for downtime.

Injection methods are recommended for those who want fast, targeted effects on deeper skin layers, while non-injection methods suit clients seeking a gradual improvement in skin tone, texture, and hydration without invasive procedures.

Innovations In Mesotherapy Application Tools And Technology

Mesotherapy has evolved significantly with innovations in tools and technology, making it safer, more precise, and accessible. Automated injection devices now allow practitioners to deliver micro-injections with accurate depth control, reducing discomfort and minimizing the risk of bruising. These tools enhance treatment consistency and enable practitioners to treat large areas more efficiently, perfect for those seeking broader skin rejuvenation.

Dermapen devices are another advancement, offering an automated version of derma rollers that allows for a more consistent needling pattern and depth control, enhancing collagen production while reducing recovery time.

For no-needle methods, advancements like ultrasound and laser-assisted delivery systems provide deeper penetration, allowing products to reach mid-dermal layers without breaking the skin. Such innovations make non-invasive mesotherapy more effective, and suitable for people seeking needle-free alternatives with stronger results.

With these advancements, mesotherapy tools are becoming available for at-home use with built-in safety features and simplified controls. Home-use derma rollers with limited needle depth and portable no-needle devices with pre-set modes make it easier to perform safe and effective mesotherapy at home. Always research the device, follow hygiene protocols, and consult a professional for personalized advice on choosing the most effective tool for your goals.

CHAPTER SIX

Mesotherapy Ingredients And Formulations

Mesotherapy involves injecting a tailored blend of ingredients directly into the skin's middle layer (mesoderm). These formulations are designed to address specific concerns such as hydration, skin rejuvenation, fat reduction, or hair growth. Typical ingredients include vitamins, amino acids, plant extracts, enzymes, and hyaluronic acid. The precise mixture depends on the treatment goal, ensuring targeted and effective delivery.

Personalized mesotherapy formulations are developed after consulting a professional who evaluates the patient's skin type, medical history, and desired outcome.

For instance, a person with dull skin might receive a vitamin C-rich solution, while those seeking anti-aging benefits might require a collagen-boosting peptide blend. Combining several active ingredients enhances the overall effect but must be done carefully to avoid adverse reactions.

The quality and sourcing of ingredients are crucial for safe and effective mesotherapy. Products should be certified, sterile, and ideally sourced from reputable pharmaceutical companies.

Misuse of unapproved products can lead to complications such as infections or allergic reactions. To ensure safety, always check for official product approvals and expiration dates before treatment.

Common Ingredients For Skin Brightening, Hydration, And Anti-Aging

For skin brightening, common mesotherapy ingredients include vitamin C, glutathione, and kojic acid. These help reduce pigmentation, even out skin tone, and restore radiance. Vitamin C boosts collagen production and offers antioxidant protection, while glutathione detoxifies and inhibits melanin production.

Hyaluronic acid is widely used for hydration because of its ability to retain moisture in the skin, improving elasticity and softness. It works well for those experiencing dryness or fine lines. Anti-aging formulations often include peptides, coenzymes, and retinol to stimulate collagen and elastin production, which enhances firmness and reduces wrinkles.

A typical treatment session involves micro-injections into the targeted area using a fine needle or mesotherapy gun. The process is generally painless, though mild redness or swelling may occur. It is essential to complete multiple sessions (usually 4 to 6) spaced two to three weeks apart for optimal results.

Fat-Burning Agents And Their Roles In Body Contouring

Mesotherapy for body contouring uses fat-dissolving agents such as phosphatidylcholine, deoxycholic acid, and L-carnitine. Phosphatidylcholine breaks down fat cell membranes, making it easier for the body to eliminate fat naturally. Deoxycholic acid, an FDA-approved compound, dissolves stubborn fat deposits, particularly under the chin and jawline.

L-carnitine promotes fat metabolism by transporting fatty acids into cells for energy production, making it popular in formulations aimed at reducing cellulite. These ingredients are injected into targeted fat pockets, such as the abdomen, thighs, or upper arms, for localized slimming.

Body contouring through mesotherapy is not a weight-loss solution but a way to target small areas resistant to diet and exercise. Multiple sessions are needed to see visible results, with a healthy lifestyle essential for maintaining outcomes.

The patient may experience mild soreness or swelling post-treatment, which usually subsides within a few days.

Understanding Personalized Formulations

Personalized mesotherapy formulations are essential for achieving optimal outcomes since everyone's skin type and treatment goals are unique. The process begins with a detailed consultation, where the practitioner assesses the patient's concerns, lifestyle, and medical history. A blend of active ingredients is then developed to address specific needs, such as hydration, anti-aging, or fat reduction.

For example, someone struggling with acne scars might benefit from a mix of hyaluronic acid, peptides, and antioxidants. On the other hand, individuals seeking hair restoration may receive formulations containing vitamins, amino acids, and DHT blockers like finasteride.

Personalization ensures that the right combination of ingredients works synergistically for the best possible effect.

The formulation may be adjusted during the course of treatment based on the patient's response. It's crucial to work with experienced practitioners who understand both dermatology and pharmacology, as incorrect formulations can cause irritation or uneven results.

Importance Of Quality And Sourcing In Mesotherapy Products

Quality control is critical when selecting mesotherapy products to ensure safety and effectiveness. Poor-quality or counterfeit products can lead to infections, allergic reactions, or inconsistent results.

Certified and pharmaceutical-grade ingredients should always be used to minimize risks.

Reliable practitioners source their ingredients from trusted pharmaceutical companies and verify batch numbers, manufacturing dates, and sterility. It's also essential that products have been tested for biocompatibility, ensuring they won't trigger adverse immune responses once injected into the skin.

Patients can ask their practitioners about the origin of the products and whether they meet regulatory standards. Using products approved by health authorities helps ensure consistent quality. Always avoid treatments from unqualified providers who cannot verify the safety or legitimacy of their formulations.

Guidelines On How To Read And Interpret Ingredient Lists

Understanding mesotherapy ingredient lists can help patients make informed decisions. Look for active ingredients like vitamins (A, C, E), peptides, and hyaluronic acid listed near the top, as these should be present in higher concentrations. Avoid products with unfamiliar fillers or allergens that may irritate.

Check for preservatives such as phenoxyethanol or parabens, which are used to prevent contamination but should be within safe limits. It's also essential to verify the absence of harmful additives, particularly for sensitive skin. Labels with terms like "sterile" or "pharmaceutical-grade" indicate higher-quality products.

Patients should consult their practitioner for clarity on any ingredient they don't understand. It's also helpful to research individual components and their benefits to verify they align with treatment goals. This step ensures transparency and builds trust between the patient and the provider.

CHAPTER SEVEN

Preparing For A Mesotherapy Session

Preparing for a mesotherapy session is essential for achieving the best results and minimizing potential risks. A week or two before your session, it's recommended to avoid blood-thinning medications or supplements like aspirin, fish oil, and vitamin E, as they can increase the chance of bruising. Refrain from consuming alcohol and caffeine 24 hours before your treatment to reduce the likelihood of swelling and discomfort. Staying hydrated is also crucial as it helps your skin recover faster.

Ensure your skin is well-prepped on the day of the procedure by cleansing it thoroughly to remove oils, makeup, and dirt. Avoid applying creams, lotions, or any products that may interfere with the mesotherapy injections. Wearing comfortable clothing is advisable, especially if your session involves multiple body areas, as this can make the experience more relaxed and convenient.

Lastly, get a good night's sleep to keep your body calm and prepared. Rest can help with pain tolerance, while a balanced diet can boost skin health, improving the treatment outcome.

Taking these preparatory steps ensures that both your skin and body are in their best possible state to receive mesotherapy effectively.

What To Expect During A Consultation

Your initial consultation for mesotherapy is where you'll discuss your goals, medical history, and expected results. The practitioner will evaluate your skin, discuss your aesthetic concerns, and recommend the best treatment plan tailored to your needs. This is also a good opportunity to understand the types of injections that will be used, such as hyaluronic acid, vitamins, or specific medications designed to achieve your desired results.

The practitioner will likely conduct a brief skin analysis to determine any sensitivities and assess how your skin might react to the treatment. They may take before photos to track progress over time. This evaluation phase helps set realistic expectations and gives you a better idea of how many sessions may be required for optimal results, depending on the targeted area and your skin's condition.

Finally, your practitioner will go over the potential risks and side effects to ensure you're fully informed. They'll provide detailed aftercare instructions and answer any specific concerns you may have. This consultation stage is key to building trust, clarifying doubts, and ensuring a smooth experience with mesotherapy.

Pre-Treatment Do's And Don'ts

In the days leading up to your mesotherapy appointment, follow specific do's and don'ts to prepare your skin and body. Do keep your skin hydrated, as well-moisturized skin responds better to treatment and aids in recovery. Do follow a gentle skincare routine; avoid exfoliating or using any active ingredients that may cause skin irritation.

On the don't side, avoid sun exposure or tanning beds for at least a week before your appointment to reduce the risk of post-treatment pigmentation issues. Skip activities that could thin your blood, such as heavy exercise, and steer clear of alcohol for 24 hours before the procedure, as it can increase the risk of bruising and swelling.

Lastly, avoid wearing makeup on the day of your session to give the practitioner a clean canvas to work with. Following these dos and don'ts can reduce potential side effects and ensure your skin is prepared for mesotherapy, maximizing the overall results and minimizing discomfort.

Questions To Ask Your Practitioner

Asking the right questions during your mesotherapy consultation is key to making informed decisions. Start by asking about their qualifications, training, and experience with mesotherapy specifically. Understanding their background will help you feel more comfortable with their expertise and give you confidence in the quality of care you'll receive.

Inquire about the ingredients in the injections and why each component is chosen for your treatment plan. Knowing the specifics will help you understand how the different vitamins, enzymes, or medications target your skin concerns.

Additionally, ask about potential side effects and the typical recovery timeline to prepare adequately for post-treatment.

Don't forget to ask about the expected number of sessions and the approximate costs involved. While some results can be seen after one session, others may require multiple treatments. Knowing this upfront can help you plan accordingly. A good practitioner will welcome your questions and provide transparent, thorough answers to address any concerns.

How To Manage Anxiety Or Discomfort Before Treatment

Feeling anxious before mesotherapy is common, especially for first-timers. To help manage this, practice deep breathing exercises in the hours leading up to your session, which can help calm the nervous system and reduce stress. Engaging in relaxing activities such as meditation, gentle yoga, or even a warm bath can also prepare your body and mind.

Distraction techniques, like listening to calming music or a favorite podcast on the way to your appointment, can also keep anxiety at bay.

Many clinics offer soothing environments with soft lighting, calming scents, and even massage chairs to help you feel at ease. Don't hesitate to bring a friend or ask if you can use headphones during the procedure to further ease your nerves.

During the consultation, let your practitioner know if you're feeling particularly nervous; they may offer a numbing cream or explain the process step-by-step to make you feel more comfortable. Communication with your practitioner can reduce anxiety and ensure you're supported throughout your treatment journey.

Understanding Cost Factors And Treatment Plans

The cost of mesotherapy can vary significantly depending on factors like the practitioner's expertise, the location of the clinic, and the type of products used in your treatment. Higher-end clinics may charge more due to their advanced equipment, premium products, and experienced staff.

Research and compare prices to get a general idea of what's reasonable for your area.

The area of treatment can also influence costs; for example, mesotherapy on the face might be less expensive than body contouring, as larger areas typically require more product and time.

Additionally, most clients need several sessions for optimal results, so inquire about packages or discounts for multiple treatments if available. Some clinics may even offer installment plans to make the process more affordable.

Your treatment plan should be tailored to your unique goals, whether targeting fat reduction, skin rejuvenation, or hair growth.

A customized plan is typically more effective and can save money in the long term by focusing only on areas that need treatment.

Knowing these cost factors allows you to budget accordingly and ensures you're investing in the best options for your needs.

CHAPTER EIGHT

Aftercare And Recovery

Key Aftercare Steps For Optimal Results

After a mesotherapy session, it's essential to follow specific aftercare practices to support healing and enhance results. Begin by avoiding touching or massaging the treated areas for at least 24 hours, as this can disturb the mesotherapy solution.

To prevent infection, keep the area clean and avoid using makeup or other skin products that could irritate.

Applying a cool compress can help soothe the skin and reduce discomfort or swelling in the first few hours after treatment.

Managing Potential Side Effects: Bruising, Redness, And Swelling

While mesotherapy is generally safe, minor side effects like bruising, redness, and swelling can occur. To manage bruising, consider using arnica gel or an arnica-based cream, which can be applied gently around the affected areas (but only if approved by your provider). Swelling can often be reduced by keeping the head elevated and sleeping on an extra pillow, allowing fluids to drain more effectively. These side effects typically subside within a few days, but if they persist, consult your practitioner.

Tips For Maintaining Results Longer

The longevity of mesotherapy results can be supported by adopting a consistent skincare routine and following a healthy lifestyle.

Drinking plenty of water aids skin hydration while avoiding sun exposure, and using a high SPF sunscreen prevents sun damage. For enhanced results, limit alcohol and tobacco, which can hinder the skin's rejuvenation process.

Additionally, gentle facial massages (as advised by your provider) a week post-treatment may improve circulation, helping maintain the skin's smooth and refreshed appearance.

Skincare Routines Post-Mesotherapy

Establishing A Gentle Skincare Routine

Post-mesotherapy, the skin is sensitive, so it's best to switch to a gentle, minimal skincare routine. For the first 24–48 hours, cleanse the face with a mild, fragrance-free cleanser and avoid exfoliants or active ingredients like retinoids and acids, as these can irritate. A hydrating moisturizer is crucial to support the skin barrier, as mesotherapy can leave the skin dry initially. Opt for products containing hyaluronic acid or ceramides to enhance moisture retention and promote a plump, hydrated look.

Adding Soothing Ingredients For Skin Recovery

Adding soothing products that contain ingredients like aloe vera, chamomile, and panthenol can help reduce redness and speed up the skin's healing process. Avoid makeup for at least 24 hours and gradually reintroduce only non-comedogenic products to prevent breakouts. Lightweight serums rich in antioxidants, such as Vitamin C, can be beneficial to combat free radicals and keep the skin glowing, but these should only be introduced a few days after mesotherapy and under professional guidance.

Long-Term Skincare Adjustments

To maintain results over time, consider a simplified, targeted skincare regimen. Incorporate regular use of SPF to protect your skin from UV rays, which can reverse mesotherapy benefits by accelerating aging signs. Weekly hydration masks can help boost moisture and maintain skin elasticity while avoiding harsh scrubs and chemical peels that can prevent irritation. Retinoids, introduced gradually after a few weeks, can further support skin texture and elasticity, but only after your provider gives the green light.

When To Schedule Follow-Up Treatments

Understanding Initial Treatment Frequency

For beginners, the initial mesotherapy treatments are often more frequent to build up and enhance results. Typically, the first four to six sessions are spaced every 1–2 weeks, depending on the targeted area and individual response.

This frequency allows the injected nutrients and vitamins to deeply penetrate and stimulate collagen production effectively. Consistency in these initial treatments establishes a good base for long-term results.

Assessing Results And Adjusting Frequency

As visible improvements develop, your practitioner may space treatments out to monthly intervals or longer. Every person's skin responds differently, so practitioners usually assess the skin's progress to decide when follow-ups are needed. If results are holding well and your skin remains firm and hydrated, treatments can often be spaced further apart, perhaps every 3–6 months. Regular check-ins help maintain your skin's radiance without overloading it with frequent injections.

Factors That Influence Follow-Up Needs

Lifestyle factors like stress, diet, hydration, and sun exposure can affect mesotherapy results, influencing how often touch-ups are needed.

People who are exposed to more environmental stressors or have naturally dry skin may benefit from slightly more frequent sessions.

Conversely, those who follow a skincare routine with sunscreen, hydration, and a healthy diet may only need periodic maintenance treatments.

CHAPTER NINE

Common Concerns And FAQS

Mesotherapy raises several common questions for beginners who want a full understanding of the procedure. This guide addresses concerns related to safety, effectiveness, expectations, and practical aspects like scheduling.

Mesotherapy involves injecting vitamins, enzymes, hormones, and other beneficial substances into the skin to rejuvenate it, targeting areas such as the face, body, and scalp for benefits like improved texture, reduced pigmentation, and enhanced hydration. Before beginning, consult with a certified practitioner to discuss any specific goals and potential risks associated with the treatment.

How Safe Is Mesotherapy, And What Are The Risks?

Mesotherapy is generally safe when administered by a licensed and experienced professional. During the procedure, tiny injections are delivered just below the skin, containing natural ingredients that are unlikely to trigger severe reactions.

Common side effects include minor swelling, redness, or bruising at the injection sites, which typically subside within a few days. Following pre- and post-treatment guidelines helps minimize risks, and practitioners often conduct a patch test to check for any allergies to ingredients.

While risks are low, patients with certain conditions, such as pregnancy, diabetes, or immune disorders, should avoid mesotherapy or consult with a healthcare provider first. The procedure's safety also depends on the hygienic standards maintained during treatment, making it essential to choose a well-reputed clinic. To further ensure safety, practitioners may also assess your skin type and any previous allergic reactions before proceeding.

Can Mesotherapy Work For Everyone?

Mesotherapy is versatile and can benefit various skin types and conditions, but results depend on individual factors like skin type, health conditions, and treatment goals. For example, individuals looking for improved skin texture, hydration, or mild fat reduction are often ideal candidates, while those with severe skin laxity may require additional or alternative treatments. Each session builds upon previous results, allowing for a gradual enhancement that naturally suits the body's rhythm of skin renewal and healing.

However, some people may experience faster results than others due to factors like age, lifestyle, and adherence to aftercare. Younger individuals with more resilient skin tend to see quicker and more pronounced changes, whereas mature skin may require more sessions to reach similar effects. By managing expectations and following the prescribed schedule, most patients find mesotherapy to be a valuable addition to their skincare routine.

Additionally, the professional administering the treatment can tailor the formula to address specific skin concerns, maximizing efficacy. Since mesotherapy is highly customizable, discussing your goals in detail during the consultation allows for a targeted approach that enhances the likelihood of satisfactory results.

Differences In Results Between Individuals

Results vary widely in mesotherapy due to individual differences in skin type, health, metabolism, and lifestyle factors. For instance, people with a fast metabolism or healthier lifestyle habits (such as hydration, a balanced diet, and good skincare) tend to see results sooner and enjoy longer-lasting effects. Skin elasticity and collagen levels also play a role; youthful skin usually shows quicker improvements, while mature skin may require more sessions to achieve desired results.

Although initial results may appear within the first few sessions, full effects often require a series of treatments over weeks or months, especially for goals like cellulite reduction or skin firming.

Each session builds on the previous, and changes typically occur subtly. It's important to remember that mesotherapy is a gradual process, so patience and consistency are key to achieving the best outcomes. Regular consultations with the practitioner allow for adjusting the treatment plan based on individual progress.

While mesotherapy is an effective standalone treatment, complementary skincare routines—like using moisturizers and sunscreens—can enhance and prolong results. For more pronounced or targeted improvements, combining mesotherapy with other treatments may also be beneficial.

What Happens If I Miss A Session?

Missing a mesotherapy session is usually not detrimental but may delay visible results since each session contributes to cumulative improvements. Typically, sessions are scheduled every one to two weeks to allow the skin to heal and respond optimally to the treatment. If you miss a session, contact your practitioner to reschedule at the nearest possible time, maintaining the recommended intervals for consistent results.

Sticking to the initial schedule is important, especially during the first few treatments, as it lays a foundation for improvements. The frequency can be modified after achieving initial goals, and maintenance sessions may be scheduled less frequently, based on individual needs. Practitioners can often provide guidance on adjusting the treatment plan without compromising effectiveness.

Should a delay occur due to unavoidable circumstances, keeping up with at-home skincare routines, hydration, and healthy habits can help sustain the results achieved so far. Returning to the planned regimen as soon as possible ensures that you continue to experience the benefits of mesotherapy in line with your aesthetic goals.

Combining Mesotherapy With Other Aesthetic Treatments

Mesotherapy can be combined with other aesthetic treatments like microdermabrasion, microneedling, or laser therapy for enhanced effects. For example, pairing mesotherapy with microneedling may amplify collagen production, improving skin texture and reducing fine lines more effectively. Discussing these options with your practitioner allows for a tailored approach that aligns with your specific skincare needs and optimizes results.

Timing is important when combining treatments; it's essential to allow adequate healing time between procedures to avoid irritation or skin overload. Often, practitioners recommend scheduling mesotherapy and other treatments like chemical peels in separate sessions, spaced out by a few weeks. This ensures each treatment can work to its full potential and that the skin has time to recover fully.

Combining mesotherapy with treatments targeting different skin layers can yield comprehensive skin rejuvenation, from improved hydration at the surface to deeper tissue remodeling. When done under professional guidance, combining aesthetic treatments helps create a balanced, natural look without overwhelming the skin.

CHAPTER TEN

Choosing The Right Practitioner And Treatment Plan

Selecting a qualified and experienced mesotherapist is crucial for the success and safety of your mesotherapy treatment. Start by researching licensed medical professionals, preferably dermatologists or plastic surgeons, who specialize in mesotherapy.

Check for certifications in cosmetic procedures and membership in recognized medical associations. It's also a good idea to ask for recommendations from friends or online reviews. Make sure the practitioner has a proven track record and can explain the entire process clearly.

Evaluating the credentials of a practitioner involves confirming their medical licenses and looking into their training in mesotherapy. Visit the clinic and assess the hygiene standards, the equipment used, and the overall environment.

The practitioner should use sterile techniques and high-quality materials. Ask about their experience specifically with mesotherapy and inquire about the potential risks involved. It's also helpful to look for before-and-after photos of previous patients to gauge their success rates.

A personalized treatment plan is essential, as mesotherapy can be tailored to various concerns such as fat reduction, skin tightening, or hair regrowth.

During your consultation, communicate your goals and discuss the number of sessions required, the substances that will be injected, and the expected outcomes.

Be realistic about what mesotherapy can achieve, as it often requires multiple sessions and results may vary. Discuss any allergies or pre-existing conditions to avoid complications, and don't hesitate to ask questions to ensure you are fully informed.

Finding A Qualified And Experienced Mesotherapist

To find a qualified mesotherapist, begin by seeking professionals with specialized training in mesotherapy. This could be a dermatologist, cosmetic physician, or plastic surgeon who has undergone additional training for this specific procedure. Certifications from recognized medical boards and specialized mesotherapy associations indicate expertise. It is also beneficial to ask for recommendations from other healthcare providers or friends who have undergone similar treatments.

When evaluating a practitioner, it's important to look beyond just their qualifications. Consider the facility where the treatment will be done.

The clinic should be clean, well-maintained, and use state-of-the-art equipment. Be sure to ask the myotherapist about their experience with your particular concern, such as fat loss or skin rejuvenation. Some professionals may specialize in specific types of mesotherapy treatments, so it's important to find someone who aligns with your goals.

Another useful tip is to set up a consultation with the practitioner. During this time, ask about their approach to mesotherapy, and how many sessions are typically needed to achieve optimal results. Feel free to ask for patient testimonials or to view before-and-after photos of previous clients. This will give you an idea of their expertise and the potential results you can expect.

How To Evaluate Practitioner Credentials And Clinic Standards

The first step in evaluating a practitioner's credentials is to verify their medical licenses and certifications. Ensure that they are trained in mesotherapy and have undergone professional courses to perform this procedure. Many reputable practitioners will display their credentials on their website or in their clinic, and you can always check with medical boards or licensing authorities to confirm their status.

In addition to credentials, clinic standards are an important factor to consider. When visiting a clinic, observe the cleanliness of the facility, the quality of the tools and equipment, and the overall ambiance. A well-maintained clinic will have high standards for patient safety and hygiene. The use of sterile equipment is vital to avoid any risk of infection or complications during the procedure.

It's also important to evaluate the practitioner's level of communication and transparency. They should be willing to explain the procedure, risks, and expected results in detail. Pay attention to how they address your concerns and whether they take the time to create a customized treatment plan for you. A responsible practitioner will focus on realistic results and ensure you understand every aspect of the treatment.

Customizing A Treatment Plan Based On Goals

Mesotherapy is highly customizable, which means your treatment plan can be specifically designed to target your unique goals. Whether you're looking to reduce fat in a particular area, rejuvenate your skin, or stimulate hair growth, your mesotherapist will tailor the treatment based on your needs.

Start by discussing your desired outcomes and any problem areas you want to address during the initial consultation. This will help the practitioner determine the appropriate injection mix and the number of sessions required.

After determining your goals, your myotherapist will outline a plan that includes the substances to be injected, which may include vitamins, enzymes, hormones, or plant extracts. They will also explain how many sessions are needed and what to expect in terms of results. For example, if you are looking to reduce cellulite, you may need multiple treatments spaced a few weeks apart.

It's important to remember that mesotherapy results are gradual and may take time to become visible. The practitioner will guide you on how to maintain the results through healthy lifestyle choices, such as diet and exercise. Be sure to communicate any medical conditions or allergies beforehand so that the treatment can be safely adjusted to suit your body.

Tips For Maintaining Realistic Expectations

One of the most important aspects of undergoing mesotherapy is maintaining realistic expectations. Mesotherapy is not a miracle cure, but it can significantly improve skin texture, reduce localized fat, or stimulate hair growth over time. During your consultation, ask your practitioner about the timeline for seeing results and the extent of the improvements you can realistically expect.

This will help you stay informed and avoid disappointment.

Remember that mesotherapy typically requires multiple sessions to achieve optimal results. Results may vary depending on individual factors like age, skin type, and the specific issue being addressed. Patience is key, as many treatments show gradual improvements over several weeks or months. It's also important to understand that while mesotherapy can enhance certain aspects of your appearance, it may not fully replace more invasive procedures like liposuction or a facelift.

Additionally, maintaining a healthy lifestyle will help extend the results of your mesotherapy treatments.

Staying hydrated, eating a balanced diet, and engaging in regular physical activity can boost the effects of the treatment. Discuss any additional steps or aftercare routines with your practitioner to ensure you get the best possible results from your sessions.

Questions To Help You Select The Right Provider

Before choosing a myotherapist, it's important to ask key questions that will help you evaluate their expertise. Begin by asking about their qualifications, certifications, and years of experience performing mesotherapy. Inquire whether they are licensed medical professionals and if they have specialized training for this procedure. Ask about their success rates with patients who have similar goals to yours, whether it's fat reduction, skin rejuvenation, or hair regrowth.

Next, ask about the specifics of the treatment. What substances will be injected, and how will the process be customized for your needs? It's also important to ask how many sessions are typically required to see results and what kind of aftercare is needed. Discuss any potential risks, side effects, and the recovery time for your particular treatment. This will help you understand what to expect and ensure that the procedure is safe for you.

Finally, make sure to ask about the costs, payment plans, and whether they offer follow-up appointments. In some cases, providers offer package deals for multiple sessions. Also, ask about any pre-treatment consultations or if you can see results from other patients. The answers to these questions will help you gauge the professionalism and transparency of the practitioner, ensuring you make an informed decision.

Conclusion

In conclusion, mesotherapy has emerged as a versatile, minimally invasive treatment with a broad range of applications in aesthetic medicine and therapeutic care. This technique, developed initially for pain management, has evolved to address diverse cosmetic concerns like skin rejuvenation, fat reduction, hair restoration, and even pigmentation irregularities. By delivering active ingredients—such as vitamins, amino acids, enzymes, and medications—directly into the middle layer of the skin, mesotherapy targets specific issues at the cellular level, often with fewer systemic side effects compared to oral or intravenous treatments.

One of the significant advantages of mesotherapy is its personalized approach. Practitioners can tailor the cocktail of ingredients to each patient's unique skin type, condition, and aesthetic goals, resulting in highly individualized treatment protocols. This customization, paired with a relatively short recovery time and a less invasive nature than traditional surgery, makes mesotherapy an attractive option for individuals seeking subtle, natural-looking improvements.

However, while mesotherapy is generally safe when performed by qualified professionals, it's not without risks. Side effects can include bruising, swelling, or infections if proper hygiene and technique are not maintained. Thus, finding an experienced, licensed practitioner is essential to minimize complications and ensure optimal results. Additionally, patients should have realistic expectations, as mesotherapy often requires multiple sessions and may not produce immediate, dramatic changes.

With advancements in the formulations used and an increasing understanding of skin physiology, the popularity of mesotherapy is likely to continue growing. For those considering the treatment, a thorough consultation can help determine if it aligns with personal health, skin condition, and desired outcomes. Overall, mesotherapy offers an innovative approach to skin and body care, bridging the gap between topical products and surgical interventions for a variety of cosmetic and therapeutic needs.

THE END

www.ingramcontent.com/pod-product-compliance
Lightning Source LLC
Chambersburg PA
CBHW052323220526
45472CB00001B/249